The Case of Cassia Essential Oils

Benefits, Properties, Applications, Studies & Recipes

by Ann Sullivan

Published in USA by:

Ann Sullivan
217 N. Seacrest Blvd #9
Boynton Beach
FL 33425

© Copyright 2015

ISBN-13: ISBN-13: 978-1544738468
ISBN-10: 1544738463

Table of Contents

Introduction

What are essential oils and how might they be used for therapeutic purposes?

Essential oils are ultra-potent oils, extracted from plants and flowers that have been utilized in medicine for centuries. Presently, they are most commonly used to supplement pharmaceutical medication, but they can also be an effective alternative to pharmaceuticals in the event that you do not have access to them. Before you dismiss essential oils as a means to support the body's natural defenses against injuries and illness, take a look at the historical evidence of the oils' medicinal competence in practice. The average age-old medical text will demonstrate that essential oils, herbs, and plenty of other natural ingredients have, for thousands of years, successfully enhanced immune function to meet and defeat any number of ailments and injuries. Though traditional medicine is considered "alternative" now, it was once the gold standard. Perhaps it still should be, as these natural age-tested remedies can fortify the body's defenses against everything from simple maladies, like headaches, cuts and bruises, to serious diseases, like cancer.

Essential oils are deemed "essential," because the oils are composed of the "essence" of the plant. The difference between essential oils and other oils – like olive oil or vegetable oil, – is that essential oils have high volatility and reduced fixation, which results in faster evaporation, enabling their popular use in aromatherapy. Even at high temperatures, olive and vegetable oils do not evaporate.

Essential oils are especially necessary when it comes to a major natural or man-made disaster or some potential viral outbreak. In these types of dire situations, you may not have quick access to standard pharmaceutical supply; so essential oils, along with other alternative medicines, will be your go-to health aids in the case of social collapse, viral outbreak, or devastating natural disaster. When medical access is null and void, alternatives to our modern-day standard are the only chance we have to keep pathogens at bay.

You probably do not realize that you already use essential oils every day. They are in perfumes, shampoos, soaps, ointments; they are even used in furniture polish. Why are they found in so many aromatic products? Essential oils are super concentrated aromatic liquids, so their scent is remarkably strong. Let's put this into perspective: to steam tea, use a few leaves of peppermint or juniper; to produce a single ounce of essential oil, five whole *pounds* of peppermint or juniper leaves are required. Some sources claim that to produce twelve pounds of essential oil would necessitate an acre of peppermint, juniper, or any other oil you are looking to produce en masse. Unlike vegetable oil, you do not often find concentrated therapeutic-grade essential oils sold in bulk; instead the oils are often sold in easily carried small, dark bottles, perfect for your GOOD bag (Get Out Of Dodge).

That is exactly what this book is aiming to help you do – get out of dodge with your most vital of essential oils intact, in particular a good supply of cassia essential oil.

Why cassia, you ask? In order to get you quickly up to speed on this most essential of oils, below we have provided a condensed synopsis of cassia, after which we will outline in greater detail the oil's history, properties, and common therapeutic uses, so that you – the consumer – might have a better understanding of the oil's benefits and applications. We have even provided supportive remedies for pure cassia, as well as blended recipes that incorporate the valuable oil. Chapter 3 will further detail past scientific research on cassia essential oil.

Now, let's get down to it – **Essential Oil 101: The Basics of Cassia.**

Summary: Cassia, or Cinnamomum cassia, is older than Moses. In fact, it was mentioned in the Bible as an ingredient amongst myrrh, cinnamon, calamus and olive oil in the Holy Anointing Oil gifted to Moses. Belonging to the cinnamon family, cassia is a "hot" oil, and is usually used in blends instead of solo. Cassia has a history in the treatment of kidney and other infections, as well as arthritis.

Description: Cassia oil is commonly extracted through steam distillation. The bark is most often used. The oil is yellow or gold in color, medium in consistency, and has a strong spicy cinnamon scent.

Uses: Beyond those applications previously

mentioned, additional uses for cassia essential oil include supporting the body's natural defenses against flu, colds, diarrhea, gas, colic, indigestion, rheumatism, arteriosclerosis, atherosclerosis, bacterial infection, immune system issues, candida, cataracts, viral infections, fungal infections, ringworm and inflammation.

Properties: Antispasmodic, antiseptic, antibacterial, antiviral, antifungal, anti-inflammatory, astringent, antidepressant, carminative, emmenagogue, circulatory, anti-emetic, anti-galactogogue, anti-rheumatic, stimulant, and febrifuge properties

Application: Dilute 1:4 with a carrier oil. You can apply topically, inhale directly, diffuse, or use as a dietary supplement.

Safety Precautions: Cassia has been approved by the FDA for internal consumption and so can be used as a dietary supplement. If you have sensitive skin, dilute heavily and test before extensive use. Do not use if pregnant.

Fun facts: The term "Cassia" is a derivative of the Hebrew word "quddah," which means "amber." The Hebrew word "quetsioth" also means "bark like cinnamon."

Being that Cassia is mentioned in the Bible, it should not come as a surprise that it also appears in the Ebers papyrus, an ancient medical record composed of 877 prescriptions and medical recipes.

Chapter 1:
Benefits of Cassia Essential Oil

Cassia oil offers a number of therapeutic benefits; but you may be wondering what these benefits are. In this chapter, we will take a closer look at the history of cassia and its many uses.

Cultivation of Cassia

Cassia essential oil, or cinnamomum cassia, is known as Chinese cinnamon, as it originates in southern China and in other countries throughout southern and eastern Asia, such as Indonesia, Malaysia, Thailand, Taiwan, Laos, Vietnam, and India. These regions cultivate the evergreen tree mainly for the species' aromatic bark, which is used in the making of essential oil, and in the making of the spice.

Closely related to Indonesian cinnamon (C. burmannii), Ceylon cinnamon (C. verum), and Vietnamese cinnamon/Saigon cinnamon (C. loureiroi), the bark of all four relatives serve as spices. The bark of Chinese cassia however, is rougher, thicker, and generally harder to crush than that of Ceylon cinnamon.

The cassia tree can reach a height of 10-15 meters, with leaves 10-15 centimeters long. The bark of the tree is hard and grey; the leaves have a red tint when they are young. The buds of the tree have also been long used in Indian spice making, and even found their way over to ancient Rome. Nowadays, Chinese cassia is the most often used cinnamon in the States.

A History of Cassia

Presently, China and Vietnam are the largest producers of Chinese cassia. Vietnam was the largest global producer of Saigon cinnamon until war interrupted production in the 1960s. The oil content and flavor of Saigon cinnamon is stronger than that of Chinese cinnamon. The war ushered Indonesian cinnamon to the forefront to fill the void of the Saigon product. Indonesian cinnamon however, has the lowest oil content, the weakest flavor, and the cheapest cost. Chinese cassia falls somewhere in the middle – lower oil content, like Indonesian cinnamon, but with a mildly sweeter flavor, close to Saigon cinnamon.

Due to this sweet flavor, cassia bark is used to flavor sweets, such as pastries, confectioneries, and other desserts, as well as meats and curries. The bark may be powdered, or used in "stick," or "quill" form. Cassia sticks are much tougher and harder than Ceylon cinnamon sticks. However, whereas Ceylon is formed into several thin layers, cassia is composed of a single thick stick and cannot be as easily ground by a spice, or coffee grinder.

The buds of cassia are only infrequently used, and they appear like cloves with a flavor similar to cinnamon. Sometimes these buds are used in the making of tea, marinade, and in the process of pickling.

Chemical Components

In order to generate the essential oil from the cassia tree, the bark, twigs, and leaves must be steam distilled. This results in the oil's key chemical components, which are primarily cinnamic aldehyde, cinnamyl acetate, chavicol, linalool, and benzaldehyde.

Main Properties of Cassia Essential Oil

Along with the properties previously mentioned in the introduction, cassia oil possesses antispasmodic, antiseptic, antibacterial, antiviral, antifungal, anti-inflammatory, astringent, antidepressant, carminative, emmenagogue, circulatory, anti-emetic, anti-galactogogue, anti-rheumatic, stimulant, and febrifuge properties. With such a versatile range, cassia is well equipped to fight off any pathogen in the body.

Cassia is composed of cinnamaldehyde, cinnamyl acetate, chavicol, linalool, and benzaldehyde. These components are what instill the enormously beneficial properties within cassia essential oil. We will outline these properties below.

Antispasmodic

The antispasmodic properties of cassia oil make it beneficial to such health issues as chronic coughing and other respiratory conditions, along with surgical processes, such as colonoscopy and gastroscopy.

Antibacterial

Cassia's antibacterial properties make it a powerful protectant against diseases produced by bacteria, such as skin issues and infections, like urinary tract or colon infections. What is great is that, unlike some prescription drugs, cassia has no ill effects on bodily health, or on the healthy natural flora that exists within the stomach and intestines.

Antiseptic

The antiseptic and disinfectant properties of cassia essential oil can be reaped topically, applied directly to wounds, or aromatically. Internal use will help keep the wounds from becoming infections, while external use will inhibit tetanus.

Antifungal

While bacteria and viruses are plenty evil, fungi commonly lead to the deadliest infections, whether external or internal. Your ears, throat, and nose are the most likely to become infected by fungi, the infections of which can be both excruciating and unsightly. If left untreated fungal infections can kill, as they may spread to the brain. Cassia essential oil protects against these infections and more.

Antiviral

The antiviral protection that cassia grants will essentially empower the immune system, building up a tougher wall of security that most colds, measles, or mumps are unlikely to scale. By boosting white blood cell count and function, this immune stimulant will ensure that your body is better prepared to protect against deadly viral infections.

Anti-inflammatory

External or internal inflammation can be reduced through the use of cassia essential oil. For instance, if you or your patient has swollen fingers from arthritis or a swollen knee from a sport's injury, oral application of cassia essential oil may decrease irritation or redness, while also soothing the pain that accompanies inflammation

Astringent

For those who do not know what an astringent is, it is a chemical compound that shrinks body tissues, which means it can aid skin issues and irritations, everything from acne to insect bites. The astringent property of cassia essential oil benefits everything from skin and hair to gums, muscles, and intestines. As an astringent, cassia is an anti-agent, combating muscle loss through the ability to strengthen. This astringent and coagulant properties also mean that diarrhea can be relieved through use of cassia essential oil, as well as bleeding from wounds and cuts.

Antidepressant

When it comes to psychological issues, the uplifting scent of cassia combats negative thoughts and supports relief from depression.

Carminative

By supporting the reduction of excess gas buildup and/or removal of gas from the intestines, cassia essential oil provides relief from abdominal pain, excess sweating, and uncomfortable indigestion.

Emmenagogue

No need to look this one up. An emmenagogue is a menstrual stimulant for those with irregular menses. Cassia regulates hormones, which means that this emmenagogue can also delay and/or reduce the symptoms of menopause, which include hormonal and mood imbalance.

Circulatory

Blood circulation is stimulated through the use of cassia essential oil. Proper blood circulation distributes oxygen and nutrients to all areas of the body, improving organ function and overall health.

Antiemetic

An anti-emetic is that which helps relieve nausea and cease vomiting. The scent of cassia provides this relief, easing these feelings of nausea and thereby alleviating the need to vomit. Great for those who have motion sickness.

Antirheumatic

Cassia's stimulant and circulatory properties contribute to its enhancing the body's healing of rheumatic and arthritic pain, as well as symptoms resulting from inflammation issues. Cassia stimulates blood circulation, warming the joints and helping to alleviate the pain.

Stimulant

Cassia is simply a stimulant. Not only does this oil stimulate the circulatory system, it also stimulates the metabolism and the nervous system, which means higher brain function, making the user more alert and active.

Febrifuge

A febrifuge is a substance that relieves fever. As cassia stimulates the circulatory system, it gives the body's immune system a leg up and, as an antiviral agent, cassia aids the body's natural defenses in fighting off infections which cause fever.

Common Medicinal Uses

A spice that has seen some history, from the days of Moses right down through present day, the therapeutic uses of cassia essential oil have accumulated a decent amount of rich history as well. This "hot" oil is most often used in blends instead of solo and has been applied on down the line to support the body's natural functions in fighting infection, and particularly in its warming relief of painful joints. Below, we will add to that list the major uses for cassia essential oil.

Diarrhea Supplement

This digestive agent is also an anti-diarrheic; that is, it supports the improvement of bowel dysfunction, helping to eliminate diarrhea. Cassia's ability to do so stems from its high fiber content and its antimicrobial properties, which both solidify the stool and help destroy the bacteria that causes diarrhea.

Combat Depression

Cassia essential oil has long been used as an uplifting mood enhancer. When it comes to psychological issues, the scent of cassia can support relief from depression and other negative feelings, such as anxiety or grief. Regular diffusion of cassia essential oil throughout the home can help trigger positivity.

Motion Sickness

For those prone to motion sickness, cassia oil may be for you. The scent of cassia eases feelings of nausea and supports the body in curtailing vomiting. If you are preparing yourself for a cross-country road trip, or have a big cruise coming up, stocking up on cassia essential oil will be a lifesaver when motion sickness throws you overboard.

Blood Circulation

Cassia's warming effect produces major responses in the body, among them increased blood circulation. When the oil vapor touches the olfactory nerve ends the pulse quickens and blood circulates, providing more oxygen to the body's organs and brain, which promotes cognitive function. The oxygenation to the brain also serves to protect against dementia, Alzheimer's, and other neurodegenerative diseases. Diabetics and arthritis, as well, are served by this boost in blood circulation.

Immune System Booster

Cassia is a superb immune system support which boosts circulation and increases white blood cell count. The oil's chemical components deliver incredible antifungal, antibacterial, and antiviral properties, making it akin to an immune shield braced to fight off angry viral strains. With such strong armor, this immune stimulant will ensure that your body is better prepared to protect against deadly viral infections.

Rheumatoid Arthritis

Those suffering from the pain and inflammation of rheumatoid arthritis can ease both through the use of cassia essential oil. Cassia's stimulant and circulatory properties contribute to enhancing the body's healing of rheumatic and arthritic pain, as well as those symptoms resulting from inflammation issues. By stimulating the blood's circulation cassia warms sore joints, relieving the pain.

Menstrual Issues

Women can benefit from administering cassia essential oil if they commonly experience painful, irregular periods, or unpleasant premenstrual symptoms. Applying cassia can help young women become regular, relieve painful menstrual cramps, and combat unpleasant attributes of PMS by better maintaining mood balance.

Safety Precautions & Common Applications

Safety

Some adverse effects may evolve when using pure essential oils. Some essential oils should not be used when pregnant. Allergic reactions may occur, especially when applied topically. Always administer an allergy test before committing fully to topical application. When used with other medications, essential oils may react negatively. If you are on any current prescription medications, or have a chronic illness such as high blood pressure, epilepsy, or liver disease, then researching the effects of essential oils against your own personal medical history will eliminate any potentially problematic issues.

Cassia has been approved by the FDA for internal consumption and so can be used as a dietary supplement. If you have sensitive skin, dilute heavily and test before extensive use. Do not use if pregnant. When applying topically, dilute cassia essential oil in a 1:4 ratio with a carrier oil. You can also inhale directly, diffuse, or use as a dietary supplement.

Blends

Oftentimes, essential oils are manufactured as blends of several pure oils. For instance, the Protective Essential Oil Blend is a mix of cinnamon, clove, rosemary, and eucalyptus. This blend can be used to boost the immune system to help support the body's natural defenses against colds, viruses, and flus. The downside to blends is that the more oils added to the mix, the higher the probability the patient may react negatively to the blend if he/she is prone to allergies. There is also the possibility of phototoxicity when working with blends.

Regardless of these possible effects, essential oils are a viable option for supporting the body's defenses against a number of conditions. Those looking to enhance the maintenance of their own personal health, or that of their families, should become educated on the uses of essential oils, their natural remedies, and the methods of application. Only then can you begin building your kit of essential oils for survival.

Chapter 2:
Recipes for Cassia Essential Oil

In this chapter, we will offer various recipes for cassia essential oil; both for pure cassia applications and blends. For pure supportive remedies, we have provided the appropriate application and dosage to help your body's natural function address specific ailments, from colds to viral infections. When it comes to blends, herbalists and aromatherapists often combine cassia essential oil with black pepper, rosemary, balsam, coriander, chamomile, ginger, nutmeg, frankincense, geranium, and some citrus oils. We will offer some fantastic supportive blending options in the second half of this chapter.

Pure Supportive Remedies

Antiseptic

To take advantage of cassia's antiseptic qualities, dilute in a 1:4 ratio with a carrier oil and apply topically to the reflex points of the feet.

Colds

Combat colds by diffusing cassia essential oil throughout the home or by placing several drops in your wet laundry before drying. If you prefer inhalation therapy, steam two drops of cassia essential oil in a pan of water, remove the steaming pan from the stove, pour into a bowl, place a towel over your head and inhale. You can also apply topically by diluting cassia in a 1:4 ratio with a carrier oil and massaging into the chest and/or the soles of the feet. Lastly, you can take cassia internally by placing a drop in your drinking water.

Digestion

To aid digestion, place a drop in your drinking water, or incorporate into your cooking. You can also apply topically by diluting cassia essential oil in a 1:4 ratio with a carrier oil and massaging it into the abdomen, as well as into the reflex points of the feet before each meal.

Flu

Support your body's natural defenses against the flu by diluting cassia essential oil in a 1:4 ratio with a carrier oil and massaging it into sore muscles and joints, into the reflex points of the feet, or over the abdominal area if you are experiencing diarrhea. You can also take internally, one drop in a glass of water, or diffuse throughout the home to support general health during cold/flu season.

Fungal Infections

Depending on the type of fungal infection and its location, combat it through internal, topical, or aromatic application. For instance, if you have athlete's foot, topical application of cassia essential oil diluted in a 1:4 ratio with a carrier oil may be the easiest and most direct approach. If you have an internal fungal infection, oral application would be more appropriate.

Helicobacter pylori

H. Pylori is a bacterium that causes stomach ulcers and other gastrointestinal issues. Support your body's defenses against H. Pylori by placing a drop of cassia essential oil in your drinking water and taking internally. You can also dilute cassia in a 1:4 ratio with a carrier oil and massage it over the abdominal area

Immune Stimulant

Give your immune system a leg up by regularly diffusing cassia throughout your home, especially during cold and flu season. The scent also uplifts and boosts energy. Alternatively, you can add a couple drops to your bathwater or dilute with a carrier oil and apply topically, massaging it into the soles of the feet. If you would prefer the steam method, steam two drops of cassia essential oil in a pan of water, remove the steaming pan from the stove, pour into a bowl, place a towel over your head and inhale. If you do not feel it has done its job the first time, you can reheat that same water and use it once more without adding more oil.

Inflammation

Calm inflammation and provide digestive system support by diluting 1 or 2 drops of cassia essential oil in a 1:1 ratio with a carrier oil, then apply topically, massaging it over the abdomen. You can also take the oil internally, placing one drop in your drinking water, or aromatically diffusing the oil, or inhaling directly.

Insect Repellant

Repel pesky insects by diluting cassia essential oil in a 1:4 ratio with a carrier oil and applying topically to the skin. The scent repels midges, mosquitoes, and gnats. You can also fill up a spray bottle with distilled water and add 5 drops of cassia per ounce, shake well, then apply as needed. Shake before each use.

Ringworm

Ringworm can be reduced through topical application, by diluting cassia essential oil in a 1:4 ratio with a carrier oil and massaging over the affected area twice a day. Once the ringworm is eliminated, continue the application for 3-5 days following recovery.

Viral Infections

Strengthen your body's defenses against viral infections by diluting cassia essential oil with a carrier oil in a 1:4 ratio and massaging it into the affected area, and into the reflex points of the feet. You can also place a few drops in your bathwater, or diffuse throughout the home

Blends

Alert Mist Spray

Ingredients

20 drops Patchouli Essential Oil

35 drops Cassia Essential Oil

35 drops Lime Essential Oil

110 drops Peppermint Essential Oil

4 ounces Distilled Water

Directions

Combine all ingredients in a dark colored glass spray bottle and if drowsy when driving, spray in your car to stimulate alertness. Alternatively, you can use the blended oils in a car diffuser.

Chest Congestion

Ingredients

1 drop Cassia Essential Oil

1 drop Lemon Essential Oil

1 tsp Carrier Oil

Directions

To clear up chest congestion, combine all ingredients and massage into your chest three times a day.

Diabetes

Ingredients

8 drops Cassia Essential Oil

8 drops Clove Essential Oil

10 drops Thyme Essential Oil

15 drops Rosemary Essential Oil

2 ounces V-6

Directions

To help maintain insulin levels, combine all ingredients and apply topically to feet and over pancreas.

Energy Booster

Ingredients

10 drops Orange Essential Oil

10 drops Cassia Essential Oil

10 drops Black Pepper Essential Oil

Directions

Diffuse blend throughout your home to stimulate energy.

Fungal Infections

Ingredients

3 drops Grapefruit Essential Oil

2 drops Cassia Essential Oil

1 drop Basil Essential Oil

1 drop Patchouli Essential Oil

½ ounce Carrier Oil

Directions

To combat fungal infections, combine all ingredients and apply topically to affected area.

Gluten Intolerance

Ingredients

1 drop Cassia Essential Oil

2 drops Grapefruit Essential Oil

2 drops Ginger Essential Oil

2 drops Lemon Essential Oil

Instructions

To help support gluten intolerance, place all ingredients into a "00" capsule, and ingest 1 capsule a day.

Immune-Boosting Spray

Ingredients

4 ounces Distilled Water

60 drops Ginger Root Essential Oil

20 drops Cassia Essential Oil

Directions

Combine all ingredients in a dark colored glass spray bottle and during cold/flu season, or if there is illness in the house, spray in all rooms to stimulate the immune system.

Immune-Boosting Topical Blend

Ingredients

5 drops Rosemary Essential Oil

8 drops Eucalyptus Essential Oil

10 drops Cassia Essential Oil

18 drops Lemon Essential Oil

20 drops Clove Essential Oil

Directions

Combine all ingredients in a dark colored bottle and during cold/flu season, or if there is illness in the house, apply topically with a carrier oil to stimulate the immune system.

Poison Ivy

Ingredients

2 drops Cassia Essential Oil

2 drops Thyme Essential Oil

13 drops Lemongrass Essential Oil

15 drops Rosemary Essential Oil

4 Tbsp. Carrier Oil

Directions

To relieve poison ivy rash, combine all ingredients and apply topically to affected area.

Room Disinfectant

Ingredients

6 drops Cassia Essential Oil

6 drops Pine Essential Oil

5 drops Juniper Berry Essential Oil

3 drops Clove Essential Oil

Directions

In a glass, marble, porcelain, or ceramic aroma lamp, combine the essential oils with water. Diffuse the oils and deeply breathe in the vapors.

Stress-Reducing Massage Oil

Ingredients

1 Tbsp. Carrier Oil

1 drop Lavender Essential Oil

3 drops Cassia Essential Oil

3 drops Grapefruit Essential Oil

4 drops Fennel Essential Oil

4 drops Roman Chamomile Essential Oil

5 drops Melissa Essential Oil

Directions

In a small bowl or jar, combine oils mixing until evenly distributed. Massage the oil into the shoulders, back, and neck. Recommended for two-time use before a stressful event, 6 hours apart to help relieve anxiety.

Uplifting Blend

Ingredients

1 drop Ginger Essential Oil

2 drops Clove Essential Oil

2 drops Cassia Essential Oil

3 drops Cardamom Essential Oil

Directions

Diffuse blend throughout your home to promote good mood and energy.

Vapor Rub

Ingredients

½ cup Olive Oil

2 Tbsp. Beeswax Pellets

20 drops Peppermint Essential Oil

20 drops Eucalyptus Essential Oil

10 drops Cassia Essential Oil

10 drops Rosemary Essential Oil

Directions

Combine ingredients in a mason jar and place jar in a saucepan with 1 inch of water. Over medium-low heat, mix beeswax and olive oil, until melted and well blended. Remove from the stove and add in the essential oils, mixing until combined. Let cool completely before use. To apply, simply rub over chest, as you would a vapor rub.

Chapter 3:
Cassia Essential Oil Studies

Many studies have been done on essential oils to discover and prove their therapeutic qualities. In the case of the great number of cassia studies, many of the properties attributed to the essential oil (noted in this book and elsewhere) are quite often validated through the scientific research of accredited universities and published by accredited scientific journals. In this chapter, we will discuss a small portion of these studies. It is important to note that research on essential oils is constantly evolving. Keep up with any recent research, as it may turn up even further valuable uses of these miracle oils.

Study 1 – Anti-inflammatory Properties

In this study published by the *Journal of Advanced Pharmaceutical Technology & Research*, the anti-inflammatory effects of cassia essential oil were examined, with the following results: "Cassia oil (CO) from different parts of Cinnamomum cassia have different active components. Very few pharmacological properties of cassia leaf oil have been reported. This study investigated and compared effects of cassia leaf oil and cinnamaldehyde on lipopolysaccharide (LPS)-activated J774A.1 cells. These results demonstrated that inhibitory effects of cassia leaf oil from C. cassia mainly came from cinnamaldehyde. This compound not only inhibited inflammatory mediators but also activated anti-inflammatory mediators in LPS-activated J774A.1 cells. It may also have an effect on iron regulatory proteins in activated macrophages."

In this study, oil was extracted from the cassia leaf to examine the effects of its volatile compositions, and in particular cinnamaldehyde, which is the organic compound that provides cassia its scent, flavor, and which has also been shown to be an anticancer and antimicrobial agent. The oil itself, and cinnamaldehyde on its own, were tested on LPS-activated J774A.1 cells – cells for which inflammation had been induced.

Both of the oils inhibited inflammation by decreasing expression of those enzymes that induce inflammation, such as nitric oxide synthase, cyclooxygenase-2, microsomal prostaglandin-E synthase-1; and by increasing expression of anti-inflammatory cytokines IL-10. Moreover, they increased the expression of Fpn1, which is a protein that transports iron from the inside to the outside of a cell.

The study demonstrates the anti-inflammatory effects of cassia essential oil, and the oil's potential in enhancing the body's natural defenses against inflammation.

Reference:
http://www.ncbi.nlm.nih.gov/pubmed/25364694]

http://www.ncbi.nlm.nih.gov/pmc/articles/PMC4215479/

Study 2 – Antifungal Properties

In this study published by *PLOS One*, the antifungal effects of cassia essential oil were examined, with the following results: "Antifungal activity of Allium tuberosum (AT), Cinnamomum cassia (CC), and Pogostemon cablin (Patchouli, P) essential oils against Aspergillus flavus strains 3.2758 and 3.4408 and Aspergillus oryzae was tested at 2 water activity levels (aw : 0.95 and 0.98)...Results of the study represent a solution for possible application of essential oil of C. cassia in different food systems due to its strong inhibitory effect against tested Aspergillus species. In real food system (table grapes), C. cassia essential oil exhibited stronger antifungal activity compared to cinnamaldehyde."

Aspergillus flavus is a pathogenic fungus appearing in cereal grains, tree nuts, and legumes, during stages of harvest, transit, or storage. Many Aspergillus flavus strains produce compounds called mycotoxins, which are toxic when consumed. A. flavus can also produce opportunistic human pathogens, causing aspergillosis, which may result in tuberculosis, or ear, eye, nose, and nail infection in immunocompromised individuals. Aspergillus oryzae is a mold that is used to ferment soybeans and alcoholic beverages in East Asian cultures.

The study showed that cassia essential oil inhibited both strains at 250 ppm and suppressed colony growth at all concentrations. These results indicate that cassia essential oil may serve a potential antifungal application in food systems against these two branches of fungi.

Reference:
http://www.ncbi.nlm.nih.gov/pubmed/23647469]

Study 3 – Insect Repellent

In this study, available on PubMed, the repellent properties of cassia essential oil were examined, with the following results: "Leptotrombidium pallidum (Nagoya, Miyagawa, Mitamura & Tamiya) is a primary vector of Orientia tsutsugamushi (Hyashi), the causative agent of scrub typhus. An assessment is made of the repellency to L. pallidum larvae (chiggers) of cassia bark, eucalyptus, and star anise oils and major constituents (E)-cinnamaldehyde, 1,8-cineole, and (E)-anethole of the corresponding oils...In the light of global efforts to reduce the level of highly toxic synthetic repellents, the three essential oils and their major constituents described merit further study as potential bio-repellents for the control of L. pallidum populations."

Leptotrombidium pallidum is endemic to Japan and are mites that transmit scrub typhus to humans through their bite. Scrub typhus is caused by Orientia tsutsugamushi, a Gram-negative bacterium and parasite. Scrub typhus is similar to other forms of typhus and includes symptoms like cough, fever, muscle pain, headache, abnormal liver function, rash, and gastrointestinal issues. Progressive strains can even cause intravascular coagulation and hemorrhaging.

This study aimed to assess the efficacy of using essential oils – among them cassia – as alternative repellents to simultaneously rid of the leptotrombidium pallidum larvae and reduce the use of highly toxic repellents by replacing them with more environmentally friendly alternatives. The results showed that cassia essential oil and its major constituent cinnamaldehyde, exhibited much higher potency as a repellent than did the conventional repellent. The study demonstrates the potential use of cassia essential oil as an insect repellent, particularly against leptotrombidium pallidum.

Reference:
http://www.ncbi.nlm.nih.gov/pubmed/23802452]

Study 4 – Skin Whitener

In this study published in the *International Journal of Molecular Sciences*, the skin-whitening effects of cassia essential oil were examined with the following results: "Essential oils extracted from aromatic plants exhibit important biological activities and have become increasingly important for the development of aromatherapy for complementary and alternative medicine. The essential oil extracted from Cinnamomum cassia Presl (CC-EO) has various functional properties; however, little information is available regarding its anti-tyrosinase and anti-melanogenic activities. In this study, 16 compounds in the CC-EO have been identified...These results demonstrate that CC-EO and its major component, cinnamaldehyde, possess potent anti-tyrosinase and anti-melanogenic activities that are coupled with antioxidant properties. Therefore, CC-EO may be a good source of skin-whitening agents and may have potential as an antioxidant in the future development of complementary and alternative medicine-based aromatherapy."

This study identified cassia oil's major components as cis-2-methoxycinnamic acid (43.06%) and cinnamaldehyde (42.37%). The study analyzed the effects of cassia essential oil and cinnamaldehyde on B16 melanoma cells and found that cassia managed to reduce the melanin content and tyrosinase activity of the cells and also reduce tyrosinase expression without demonstrating cytotoxicity.

The results of this study showcase the oil's antioxidant activities at their best and also demonstrate the anti-tyrosinase and anti-melanogenic properties of the oil, which give it potential as a skin-whitening agent.

Reference:
http://www.ncbi.nlm.nih.gov/pubmed/24051402]

http://www.ncbi.nlm.nih.gov/pmc/articles/PMC3794828/pdf/ijms-14-19186.pdf]

Study 5 – Antifungal Properties

In this study, available on PubMed, the antifungal effect of cassia essential oil was examined, with the following results: "The inhibitory effect of cassia oil alone or in combination with calcium chloride (CaCl2) against Alternaria alternata in vitro and in vivo was assessed on cherry tomatoes...The results indicated that cassia oil alone or in combination with CaCl2 significantly enhanced defense-related enzyme activities, such as peroxidase and polyphenol oxidase. Together, these data suggest that the combination of cassia oil and CaCl2 may be an efficient method to limit cherry tomato decay caused by fungi."

Alternaria alternata is a fungus which causes leaf spots and a variety of other plant diseases in more than 380 plant species. The opportunistic pathogen can also result in asthma and upper respiratory infections in humans, especially those with compromised immune systems.

The results of the study demonstrated that when combined with calcium chloride, cassia essential oil's inhibitory effects on the growth of A.alternata increased. The combination of 500 µl of cassia oil per liter and 0.25% calcium chloride demonstrated significant inhibition on decay in the cherry tomato. Even better, the quality of the tomatoes was not affected by these treatments, which indicates that this cassia-calcium chloride combo may be an effective antifungal in the preservation of fruit and vegetables affected by alternaria alternata.

Reference:
http://www.ncbi.nlm.nih.gov/pubmed/24215690]

Study 6 – Antibacterial/Antifungal

A study, available on PubMed, examined the antibacterial and antifungal effects of cassia essential oil, with the following results: "Both Cinnamomum verum J.S. Presl. and Cinnamomum cassia Blume are collectively called Cortex Cinnamomi for their medicinal cinnamon bark. Cinnamomum verum is more popular elsewhere in the world, whereas C. cassia is a well-known traditional Chinese medicine. An analysis of hydro-distilled Chinese cinnamon oil and pure cinnamaldehyde by gas chromatography/mass spectrometry revealed that cinnamaldehyde is the major component comprising 85% in the essential oil and the purity of cinnamaldehyde in use is high (> 98%)...The antimicrobial effectiveness of C. cassia oil and its major constituent is comparable and almost equivalent, which suggests that the broad-spectrum antibiotic activities of C. cassia oil are due to cinnamaldehyde."

This study evaluated both cassia essential oil and its isolated major constituent, pure cinnamaldehyde, and found that they were equally effective in inhibiting the growth of various isolates of bacteria, fungi, and molds.

Some of the bacteria tested include Staphylococcus aureus, E. coli, and Salmonella typhimurium.

Staphylococcus aureus is Gram-positive bacterium. Although Staphylococcus aureus is part of the normal human skin flora and respiratory tract and is not typically pathogenic, those with compromised immune systems can potentially develop an infection from the bacteria. When it becomes so, S. aureus produces respiratory issues like sinusitis, skin infections, and even food poisoning. Escherichia coli is a bacterium, as well, though it is Gram negative, rather than Gram positive. E. coli can often result in serious food poisoning. Salmonella strains can cause an array of illnesses, from typhoid fever to food poisoning.

The fungi tested includes Candida strains, such as Candida albicans and Candida tropicalis, which develop as yeast and filamentous cells and can potentially cause genital and oral infections. Candida albicans also increases the probability of mortality in immunocompromised individuals (cancer or AIDS patients, for instance).

The filamentous molds tested include Aspergillus species, which are commonly found in soil, agricultural goods, marine species, and farmed animals. When consumed by humans the fungus causes chronic immunosuppressive, neurotoxic, genotoxic, and carcinogenic issues. Furthermore, the fungi's airborne spores produce asthma in kids and other lung diseases. Consequently, the ability to control this fungi is imperative to human health, animal health, and agricultural health.

The MICs of both oil and cinnamaldehyde for bacteria were similar, which indicates that much of the oil's antibacterial and antifungal activity is due to its major component, cinnamaldehyde.

Reference: http://www.ncbi.nlm.nih.gov/pubmed/16710900]

Study 7 – Anticancer

In this study published by the *National Institutes of Health,* the anticancer effects of cassia essential oil were examined, with the following results: "Colorectal cancer (CRC) is a major cause of tumor-related morbidity and mortality worldwide. Recent research suggests that pharmacological intervention using dietary factors that activate the redox sensitive Nrf2/Keap1-ARE signaling pathway may represent a promising strategy for chemoprevention of human cancer including CRC. In our search for dietary Nrf2 activators with potential chemo preventive activity targeting CRC, we have focused our studies on trans-cinnamic aldehyde (cinnamaldehyde, CA), the key flavor compound in cinnamon essential oil. Here we demonstrate that CA and an ethanolic extract (CE) prepared from Cinnamomum cassia bark, standardized for CA content by GC-MS analysis, display equipotent activity as inducers of Nrf2 transcriptional activity...Taken together our data demonstrate that the cinnamon-derived food factor CA is a potent activator of the Nrf2-orchestrated antioxidant response in cultured human epithelial colon cells. CA may therefore represent an underappreciated chemopreventive dietary factor targeting colorectal carcinogenesis."

The study examined the use of cassia essential oil's chemical compound, cinnamaldehyde, as a strategy for chemoprevention in cancer, particularly in colorectal cancer. The study found that cinnamaldehyde activated the antioxidant response in cultured human epithelial colon cells, which means cassia can indeed serve as a chemopreventive dietary factor when fighting rectal cancer.

Reference:
http://www.ncbi.nlm.nih.gov/pubmed/20657484]

http://www.ncbi.nlm.nih.gov/pmc/articles/PMC3101712/pdf/nihms293405.pdf]

Chapter 4:
The Ins & Outs of Essential Oils

Where do essential oils come from?

Plants and plant species naturally produce essential oils for various reasons; one being to draw pollinator insects to them, another being to repel invading organisms (bacteria, animals). A number of chemical compounds compose each plant's essential oil, and the combination of these compounds are specific to each oil, which then instills in the oil its own unique properties. Essential oils can be harnessed from all sorts of plant components, including flowers, leaves, bark, fruit, roots, and resin. For instance, cinnamon oil is harnessed from bark, lemon oil from the peel, and lavender oil from lavender flowers. Certain plants can produce a few chemical variants of the same essential oil, which are acquired from different parts of the plant. Some of these parts produce a large amount of oil, while others produce just a smidgen. The oil's quality and potency depends upon a number of factors, including the subspecies of the plant, its soil conditions, the time of year, and even the time of day you harvest it.

How are essential oils extracted?

Essential oils can be extracted from plants through various methods, including pressing, distillation, solvent, and maceration. Let's take a brief look at each:

Pressing Method

Commonly used with citrus fruit, the pressing method extracts the oil through a technique which involves pushing the fruit peels through a press. Oily fruits and plants are best suited for this technique. Orange oil, for example, is extracted from orange skins through the pressing method.

Distillation Method

This technique harkens back to the days of moonshiners, as the same sort of method used to create strong liquor can be used to extract essential oils. Using a still, boiled water, and plant materials, will create steam which is then cooled by coils and condensed into a combination of water and oil. This combination does not mix, so the oil can then be extracted from it.

Solvent Method

Through a multi-step process, certain plant and flower oils can be extracted using alcohol and other solvents, which extort the essential oil from the plant materials.

Maceration Method

When a "carrier," fixed oil, or lard is mixed with the plant material and set out in the sun over a period of time, the carrier oil is infused with the plant's essence. Heat sources, other than the sun, are often used to speed the process. Throughout the process more plant material is added to produce a more potent oil.

How do you use essential oils?

Although some studies about the effectiveness of essential oils are conducted by small companies or even individuals, a number of them are conducted by the food and cosmetic industries. In general, the pharmaceutical industry shows next to no interest in herbal medicine, primarily because there are few options to patent such products. As such, the product's lack of profitability results in a lack of research funding. Regardless, the historical uses of essential oils tell us what we need to know: these oils have been effectively administered for centuries. The therapeutic qualifications of essential oils can be plotted in the survival of the human race across cultures and generations.

Another reason that studies on essential oils have not resulted in much conclusive evidence as to their overall effectiveness is because definitive results are sometimes difficult to prove, as the quality of each batch of oil can vary for a number of reasons. One is that essential oils are impossible to standardize. As mentioned above, even the slightest variance in soil conditions and the time of harvesting – as well as innumerable other factors – will produce a different product quality and potency. In addition, essential oils are often obtained from various species of the same plant; Eucalyptus radiata and Eucalyptus globulus can both be used in the making of therapeutic-grade eucalyptus oil and as a result, they may have slightly different properties and degrees of strength or effectiveness.

Just as there are a number of methods by which to extract essential oils, there are a number of methods to administer them therapeutically. The variety of chemical compounds in each essential oil means that their benefits and applications also vary across the board. Below are a few of these methods.

Topical Administration

Direct application of many essential oils works like a sponge, as skin absorbs chemicals and other things (like sunlight, for instance). Topical application is best when you want to clear up an ailment on the skin's surface, or in the underlying muscle tissue. When applying topically, you may either massage the oil into the skin, or simply dab on the skin for therapeutic results. You might combine the essential oil with a carrier oil for topical use in order to dilute its potency. This is safer, as the oil is concentrated. You may support your body's defenses against rash or muscle pain in this manner, but you should always test your patient for allergies before applying. Adverse effects are produced by natural chemicals as much as synthetic ones; poison ivy, for example.

To test for allergens, place a drop or two on your patient's inner forearm. If a rash develops within 12 to 24 hours, then the patient is allergic. In addition, phototoxicity – sun exposure resulting in an exacerbated burn – may be an issue when citrus oils are applied topically. One must proceed with caution when applying essential oils using this method.

Inhalation Therapy

Commonly known as "aromatherapy," this essential oil application is effective for inner ailments, like sore throat or cold. In a steaming bowl of distilled, or sterilized water, add a few drops of essential oil and with a towel over your head, bend over the bowl and inhale. The towel captures the vapors making the technique even more effective. Essential oils can also be placed in a diffuser, or potpourri throughout a room, to produce somewhat diluted medicinal effects.

Ingestion

When using this method proceed with caution. Direct

ingestion of essential oils must be monitored and applied in small doses that are diluted in a tablespoon or more of any carrier oil – olive oil, for example. If you are unsure of dosage amounts, then make a tea with the relevant herb instead. Although the effects of this diluted use may be weaker, this application is a better alternative than an overdose of essential oils.

What are the general benefits of using essential oils?

Replacement for Prescription Drugs

One practical benefit for using essential oils is their substitutive nature; they can replace Rx drugs, which is the ultimate reason to educate yourself on their administration and to begin stockpiling your essential oil supply. One of the potential threats of economic or social collapse, is the lack of resources, and primarily the inability to procure prescription drugs. As such, finding suitable alternatives should be a priority when prepping for the worst.

Their portability is also a major bonus when it comes to survival prepping. The fact that these ultra-concentrated oils take up little-to-no space makes toting them to your shelter all the easier should the need arise. Because essential oils are highly concentrated, the application used in most methods of administration requires only a drop or two of oil, which means a tiny bottle will be long-lasting.

Cheap, but Effective Alternative

Though money may be the last thing on your mind when it comes to prepping for a survival situation (money may even be obsolete in the event of social collapse), it is worth noting that the expense of essential oils pales in comparison to prescription drugs. In fact, whether or not you are forced to survive on essential oils due to a lack of prescription reserves, in some cases, you might consider substituting your prescriptions for these inexpensive alternatives regardless. Essential oils are a cost efficient, yet equally effective alternative to prescription medicine.

No Expiration Date

Another benefit of essential oils is that they do not expire, nor do they have "proper storage" requirements. A number of medicines and medicinal products must be replaced every couple years; this sets essential oils ahead of the pack when it comes to shelf life.

Versatility

Essential oils also offer great versatility. Apart from providing health benefits, essential oils can be repurposed for household and hygienic applications. For instance, if you are looking for something that might serve your dental hygiene needs in a time of crisis, thieves oil is your go-to essential oil. If you want to maintain your skin's health, frankincense and lavender will do the trick; the latter also serves as sunscreen, so you can prevent sun damage as well.

When it comes to the house or shelter you can use essential oils to deodorize, which will come in handy in a disaster scenario where things might start to smell due to lack of proper utilities and care. For example, after the 2011 tsunami and the subsequent nuclear reactor meltdown in Japan, a nurse named Risa Nakahira used essential oils to deodorize and sanitize putrid public bathrooms in overpopulated evacuation facilities. As relief workers searched for survivors, often wading through debris and decay, Nakahira also deodorized their boots and masks using essential oils. The possibilities of these natural oils are endless.

They are also versatile when it comes to the range of patients they are capable of supporting. The health of everyone from your great grandfather to your infant baby, can be fortified with the aid of essential oils in the appropriate dosage. They even come in handy when treating livestock or pets. From teething infants to dementia in the elderly, from teenagers with acne to dogs with urinary tract infections, essential oils can serve any patient with nearly any ailment.

Conclusion

Now that you know all about what cassia essential oil can do for you – where it originates, how it is extracted, its benefits and properties, and the different methods of administration – you can use it confidently to support the body's defenses against health issues and start to assemble a kit of essential oils for survival. Essential oils can be purchased online, or at your local holistic treatment store.

The various benefits of essential oils and their properties are countless. To build your own kit, first focus on acquiring the essential oils which may bear more relevance to your health issues, or the potential health threats within your environment. In the event of a viral outbreak, for instance, cassia essential oil will be one of your more crucial oils – along with oregano, lemon, frankincense, and cinnamon (eBooks also available for purchase) – due to their antiviral and immuno-supportive properties.

Used as a supplement, or as your go-to for skin conditions, infections or immune-boosting agents, the application of cassia essential oil in medicine has survived for centuries and will survive centuries more. When it comes down to it, you do not need to rely on pharmaceuticals; essential oils, herbs, and plenty of other natural ingredients can be used to help support the body's natural function against any number of health issues, whether ailment or injury.

Essential oils are essential to your survival in the case of viral outbreak, social collapse, or natural disaster, because when the SHTF your access to pharmaceuticals will likely either be limited or eliminated altogether. Alternatives to our modern-day standard will equate survival when no other option exists. When it comes to a life-or-death situation, you cannot let your health decline, no matter the state of the world

DISCLAIMER AND/OR LEGAL NOTICES: Every effort has been made to accurately represent this book and it's potential. Results vary with every individual, and your results may or may not be different from those depicted. No promises, guarantees or warranties, whether stated or implied, have been made that you will produce any specific result from this book. Your efforts are individual and unique, and may vary from those shown. Your success depends on your efforts, background and motivation.

The material in this publication is provided for educational and informational purposes only and is not intended as medical advice. The information contained in this book should not be used to diagnose or treat any illness, metabolic disorder, disease or health problem. Always consult your physician or healthcare provider before beginning any nutrition or exercise program. Use of the programs, advice, and information contained in this book is at the sole choice and risk of the reader.